SHINGLES

An Essential Guide to Shingles: How to Get Diagnosed, Get Treatment, and Maintain Your Skin's Health for Life

CHAD BRUNO

Table of Contents

Introductory

Herpes zoster, more often known as shingles, is a painful viral infection that manifests itself in a blistering rash. The varicella-zoster virus, also responsible for chickenpox, is to blame. The chickenpox virus can lay dormant in nerve cells for years after an infection has occurred. The virus can reactivate later in life, resulting in a case of shingles.

• The first signs are usually discomfort or a burning feeling, and they can be quite intense.

• After the initial agony has subsided for a few days, a red, painful rash may form. It is characterized by fluid-filled blisters and typically manifests in a localized area on one side of the body or face. Wherever the virus has reactivated, the rash will follow the path of an affected nerve.

• The rash could cause itching.

• Some persons with shingles also experience other symptoms, such as a high temperature, a headache, extreme weariness, and photosensitivity.

If someone who has never had chickenpox or been immunized against the virus comes into close contact with the fluid from a shingles blister, they may become infected. In most cases, shingles will clear up on their own, but painkillers and antiviral drugs can help alleviate symptoms and lessen the likelihood of complications.

If the rash appears near the eye or the person has a compromised immune system, those who fear they have shingles should visit a doctor immediately. Early therapy can help minimize the duration of the sickness and lessen the risk of consequences, such as postherpetic neuralgia, which is chronic nerve pain that can remain long after the rash has healed.

CHAPTER ONE
Understanding the Significance of Shingles

Education about shingles is important for many reasons:

• Knowing the signs and potential complications of shingles might help people get medical help quickly when they develop symptoms. Pain can be lessened, the severity of the sickness mitigated, and complications prevented if therapy begins early.

• Protect yourself from shingles with the help of science and get vaccinated. The chance of getting shingles and its complications can be greatly reduced with the shingles vaccine, especially in the elderly. Awareness of the availability and importance of shingles vaccines can motivate more people, particularly those in high-risk age groups, to be vaccinated.

• People at higher risk for getting severe instances of shingles include people with weaker immune systems as a result of medical disorders or drugs. Healthcare practitioners can better identify and protect at-risk people through vaccination and early intervention if they are aware of the risks associated with shingles.

• Though the rash associated with shingles is not communicable, the varicella-zoster virus that causes it can be spread to people who have never had chickenpox or who have not been immunized against it. One way to stop the spread of shingles is to raise awareness about the dangers of touching infected blisters and the need for extreme cleanliness and caution.

• Post herpetic neuralgia (PHN) is a painful complication of shingles that can last for months or even years after the rash has gone away, and it is difficult to treat. Improved diagnosis, treatment, and prevention of long-term consequences from shingles can result from increased public awareness.

- By increasing the public's understanding of shingles and its consequences, public health agencies and healthcare organizations will be better equipped to devise methods for prevention, education, and vaccine campaigns to lessen the disease's impact.

- Pain, discomfort, and general impairment to daily life are common reactions to shingles. A higher level of understanding can encourage people to take action and get the medical attention they need to alleviate their symptoms and improve their quality of life.

In conclusion, it is crucial to raise public awareness about shingles so that the disease can be diagnosed and treated early, that vulnerable populations are protected, that transmission is reduced, that complications are managed, that public health measures are implemented, and that the quality of life of those who contract the virus is enhanced. The public health and individual health outcomes may benefit from raising awareness about shingles and its prevention.

Can Anyone Get Shingles?

Anyone who has previously been infected with the varicella-zoster virus (the same virus that causes chickenpox) is at risk of developing shingles. However, the likelihood of getting shingles varies from person to person. Herpes zoster risk factors include:

• Shingles is more common in the elderly; the risk rises sharply after age 50. The risk of shingles also appears to increase with age.

- Only those who have had chickenpox in the past are susceptible to developing shingles. You cannot get shingles if you have never had chickenpox or been immunized against it.

- People with compromised immune systems due to illness (such as HIV/AIDS), medication (such as immunosuppressants or steroids), or treatment (such as chemotherapy), are more likely to get shingles. This is because a healthy immune system plays a key role in controlling the infection.

- **Stress:** Extreme stress can suppress the immune system, making a preexisting case of shingles more likely to manifest.

• Physical Trauma, Injury, or Surgery: The stress put on the body and immune system from physical trauma, injury, or surgery can also provoke a shingles epidemic.

• Shingles occur more frequently in females than males.

• Having a history of shingles in your family may put you at a slightly higher risk of contracting the disease yourself.

• Diabetes and other chronic conditions may increase the

likelihood that you will develop shingles.

• The chance of having shingles can be greatly reduced by getting vaccinated; the vaccine is now only available for adults. Vaccination against shingles is strongly suggested by the CDC for all persons over the age of 50.

It's vital to realize that shingles is not communicable in the same way that chickenpox is. Although the varicella-zoster virus can be passed from a person with shingles to someone who has never had chickenpox or been vaccinated, the unvaccinated individual will develop chickenpox instead of shingles.

Those who are particularly worried about contracting shingles or who fall into a high-risk category should talk to their doctor so that they can receive advice on preventative and treatment measures, such as the shingles vaccination.

CHAPTER TWO
The Signs and Wonders of Shingles

Herpes Zoster (shingles) is diagnosed by looking for a set of symptoms that match a patient's history and physical examination. Here are some of the most typical signs of shingles and how to diagnose it:

Symptoms:

1. Pain: The first and generally most prominent sign of shingles is pain. It is common to characterize this discomfort as a burning, tingling, or stabbing sensation. It may come before the rash appears, and it can be fairly intense. Pain is typically confined to one side of the head, face, or body because of where the affected nerves are located.

2. Painful redness and itching appear on the skin a few days after the initial pain has started. Clusters of fluid-filled blisters make up this rash. Depending on where the damaged nerve is located, it may be isolated or spread across a greater area.

3. Itching: The rash may cause irritation, and as blisters heal, crusts may form.

4. In addition to the rash, fever, headache, exhaustion, and sensitivity to light are among possible complications of shingles.

Methods of Diagnosis:

- **Clinical Examination:** A healthcare provider will normally start by evaluating the affected area and enquiring about the symptoms. A clinical diagnosis of shingles can usually be made based on the patient's description of the discomfort and the presence of a painful rash that follows a specific nerve pathway.

- Your medical history, including any prior cases of chickenpox or shingles, will be inquired about by your doctor.

- The fluid from the shingles blisters may be collected for laboratory testing in some circumstances, such as when the diagnosis is unclear or complications are suspected. The existence of the varicella-zoster virus can be verified in this way.

If the rash appears near the eye or if you have a compromised immune system, you should visit a doctor right once if you think you have shingles. Antiviral medication administered early on helps alleviate symptoms and lessen the likelihood of problems. The severity of nerve involvement or consequences may also necessitate the use of further diagnostic procedures.

Early diagnosis and treatment can make a big difference in the intensity and length of shingles, which can be painful and irritating. A medical practitioner should be consulted for examination and treatment if you are at risk for shingles or if you are having symptoms.

CHAPTER THREE
Problems Caused by and Solutions to Shingles

Herpes zoster, also known as shingles, can have serious consequences if the symptoms are ignored or if the affected person does not receive quick treatment. Possible side effects and remedies for shingles include the following:

Complications:

• Postherpetic Neuralgia (PHN) is a painful condition that can develop after shingles infection. Nerve discomfort that lasts long after the rash from shingles has healed is called postherpetic neuralgia

(PHN). It may last a few weeks, or it may last a few years.

• Inflammation of the eye (herpes zoster ophthalmicus), corneal damage, and even permanent blindness can result if shingles spreads to the area around or into the eye. In these situations, getting medical help right away is essential.

• Infections of the SkinBlisters from shingles, or the skin around them, can become infected with bacteria, needing antibiotic treatment.

• Rarely, shingles can cause neurological complications such as encephalitis (inflammation of the brain) or myelitis (inflammation of the spinal cord).

• **Nerve injury:** Shingles can lead to injury or inflammation of the nerves, producing symptoms including muscle weakness or paralysis.

Treatments:

• Antiviral drugs, such as acyclovir, valacyclovir, or famciclovir, are the first line of defense against shingles. When administered promptly, ideally within 72 hours of the onset of symptoms, these medications can help lessen the intensity and duration of the illness.

- **Pain Management:** Over-the-counter pain medications such acetaminophen or nonsteroidal anti-inflammatory medicines (NSAIDs) can help manage the pain associated with shingles. Stronger pain drugs may be required if the pain is severe.

- Pain can be reduced by applying a topical lotion or ointment that contains a pain reliever, such as lidocaine, capsaicin, or a numbing ingredient.

- Inflammation caused by shingles can be treated with corticosteroids in some situations, particularly if the condition has spread to the eyes.

• Prescription pain relievers, antidepressants, antiseizure drugs, and topical therapies like lidocaine patches are some of the options available for managing postherpetic neuralgia.

• If shingles spreads to the eye, treatment may include antiviral eye drops or ointments, and in extreme situations, a visit to an ophthalmologist for evaluation and maybe surgery.

• **Protective Steps:** Vaccination is the best way to avoid getting shingles. The shingles vaccine is indicated for persons over 50 and can dramatically lower the risk of developing shingles.

Seek medical assistance immediately if you suspect you have shingles or if the condition worsens, especially if the affected area is close to the eye or if you have a compromised immune system. A more manageable disease and fewer complications are possible with early diagnosis and treatment. Ongoing care and pain control may be required in cases of postherpetic neuralgia and other long-term consequences.

Strategies to Reduce the Risk of Shingles

Vaccination and adopting healthier habits can significantly lower your chance of contracting shingles. To avoid getting shingles, keep these things in mind.

1. Vaccination:

• Vaccination is the best protection against shingles.

The shingles vaccination is recommended for individuals 50 and older by the Centers for Disease Control and Prevention (CDC).

• Two vaccinations exist to prevent shingles:

Shingrix, a non-live vaccination, is highly recommended. It's given in two doses, with the second one coming 2-6 months after the first, and it offers excellent protection against shingles.

In comparison to Shingrix, the effectiveness of the older live vaccine Zostavax is lower. Some people may still consider it if they can't get Shingrix or if Shingrix doesn't work for them.

2. Be sure to stick to a healthy routine:

• Having a robust immune system can be helpful in warding off shingles. A nutritious diet, regular exercise, and stress management can all help keep your immune system strong.

3. Reducing Stress:

• Some people may develop shingles because their immune systems were weakened by chronic stress. Engage in stress-reduction tactics like meditation, deep breathing exercises, and relaxation activities.

4. Clean Your Hands:

• Although the disease itself is not communicable, the fluid from shingles blisters can spread the virus to those who have never had chickenpox or been vaccinated. Maintaining proper hand hygiene is an important step in stopping the transmission of the infection.

5. Stay Away From Each Other

• If you have an active shingles rash, avoid close contact with pregnant women, those with compromised immune systems, and newborns who have not been vaccinated or have not had chickenpox.

6. Varicella-Zoster Virus Infection Treatment:

• A reduced risk of acquiring shingles in the future may result from prompt treatment of an active varicella-zoster (chickenpox) infection.

7. Treatment with antiviral medicine and quick medical attention might lessen the severity of shingles and the likelihood of complications if you contract the disease.

8. Knowledge and understanding:

• If you are in an at-risk age range, you should inform yourself and others about the dangers of shingles. Promote preventative measures such as immunization and prompt medical care for symptoms.

Because shingles may be so painful and disabling, and because consequences like postherpetic neuralgia can have a permanent influence on quality of life, it's crucial that the disease be avoided whenever possible. The chance of getting shingles and its complications can be greatly reduced by getting vaccinated. Talk to your doctor if you have questions regarding shingles vaccinations or other methods of protection.

CHAPTER FOUR
The Reality of Shingles

The pain, itching, and limited mobility that come along with shingles make daily life difficult. The following are some methods and advice for managing shingles:

1. Seek immediate medical assistance if you suspect or have been diagnosed with shingles. Antiviral therapy administered early in the course of sickness can lessen the intensity of symptoms and lessen the likelihood of consequences.

2. Managing the discomfort: Shingles discomfort is notoriously bad. Pain can be managed with over-the-counter medications such acetaminophen or nonsteroidal anti-inflammatory medicines (NSAIDs). Stronger pain drugs may be required if the pain is severe. Your doctor can provide treatment options to alleviate your pain.

3. Pain and itching can be reduced by using a topical lotion or ointment such as lidocaine, capsaicin, or a numbing ingredient.

4. You need to get some shut-eye to help your body mend. Don't push yourself too hard, and rest if you're feeling pain or discomfort.

5. Keep yourself hydrated and eat healthily to ensure optimal performance. A healthy immune system and complete recovery are both aided by eating well.

6. Stress Reduction: High stress levels might increase the symptoms of shingles. Try some deep breathing, meditation, or relaxation activities to calm down.

7. Wearing or touching anything that can exacerbate the shingles outbreak should be avoided. Comfort can be increased by wearing loose, soft garments.

8. Although shingles is not as contagious as chickenpox, it is nevertheless important to avoid coming into touch with those who have not had shingles or who have not been immunized against it.

9. If your doctor has recommended an antiviral medicine, it is important to take it exactly as advised.

10. Listen to Your Doctor: Adhere to Your Doctor's Recommendations and Treatment Plan. They may suggest a course of treatment and schedule follow-up visits.

11. Work closely with your healthcare practitioner to manage the pain and investigate treatment options, which may include prescription drugs, if you develop postherpetic neuralgia (PHN).

12. Helpful advice: lean on your loved ones for moral support. Having them around during recuperation can be a huge assistance, both practically and emotionally.

13. If you are in an at-risk age range, you may want to consider getting the shingles vaccine after you have recovered from the disease. In doing so, you can lessen your chances of contracting shingles in the future.

Although having shingles can make daily life difficult, it can be controlled with the help of medical professionals, painkillers, and emotional support from loved ones. Seek out the advice of a medical professional for specific recommendations and to deal with any issues or difficulties related to shingles.

The Signs and Wonders of Shingles

Shingles, commonly known as herpes zoster, is diagnosed by a medical professional based on the patient's presentation of the disease's characteristic symptoms. Here are some of the most typical signs of shingles and how to diagnose it:

Symptoms:

1. Pain: The first and generally most prominent sign of shingles is pain. It is common to characterize this discomfort as a burning, tingling, or stabbing sensation. It may come before the rash appears, and it can be fairly intense. Pain is typically confined to one side of the head, face, or body because of where the affected nerves are located.

2. Painful redness and itching appear on the skin a few days after the initial pain has started. Clusters of fluid-filled blisters make up this rash. Depending on where the damaged nerve is located, it may be isolated or spread across a greater area.

3. Itching: The rash may cause irritation, and as blisters heal, crusts may form.

4. In addition to the rash, fever, headache, exhaustion, and sensitivity to light are among possible complications of shingles.

Methods of Diagnosis:

1. Clinical Examination: A healthcare provider will normally start by evaluating the affected area and enquiring about the symptoms. A clinical diagnosis of shingles can usually be made based on the patient's description of the discomfort and the presence of a painful rash that follows a specific nerve pathway.

2. Your medical history, including any prior cases of chickenpox or shingles, will be inquired about by your doctor.

3. The fluid from the shingles blisters may be collected for laboratory testing in some circumstances, such as when the diagnosis is unclear or complications are suspected. The existence of the varicella-zoster virus can be verified in this way.

If you notice a rash around your eye or have a compromised immune system and fear you have shingles, consult a doctor immediately. Antiviral medication administered early on helps alleviate symptoms and lessen the likelihood of problems. Ongoing care and pain control may be required in cases of post herpetic neuralgia and other long-term consequences.

A competent medical opinion is necessary for a proper diagnosis of shingles and subsequent therapy. Early intervention can make a substantial difference in the duration and severity of the condition.

Conclusion

Reactivation of the varicella-zoster virus, also known as the chickenpox virus, causes shingles, also known as herpes zoster. Symptoms of shingles include a painful rash that breaks out in fluid-filled blisters, itching, and in some cases fever, headache, and sensitivity to light.

Clinical evaluation, in which medical professionals examine the affected area and take the patient's medical history into account, is the gold standard for diagnosing shingles. The presence of the virus can be confirmed using certain laboratory techniques, such as the collection of fluid from shingles blisters.

Postherpetic neuralgia, which can cause persistent nerve pain, is a complication that can be avoided with prompt diagnosis and treatment. Antiviral medicines and pain control are crucial components of the therapy approach.

Vaccination, healthy living, stress management, and knowledge of transmission risks are all effective ways to prevent shingles. The risk of shingles and its complications can be greatly reduced with vaccination.

Supportive care, effective pain management, and following medical advice are all essential for getting better after being diagnosed with shingles. Early intervention can significantly alter the course and severity of the illness, so it's important to see a doctor if you suspect or experience symptoms of shingles.

In sum, shingles is a condition that, with the right medical care and support, can be effectively managed, and the prevalence of the disease can be mitigated by raising awareness about prevention strategies.

THE END

www.ingramcontent.com/pod-product-compliance
Lightning Source LLC
Chambersburg PA
CBHW050704250726
48662CB00002B/833